D1242219

WARNING

Before beginning this or any exercise program consult your physician or medical professional to verify that you are healthy enough for exercise and that this program is appropriate for your specific condition. This program is intended for people with the common sources of back pain. It is possible that you have a variety of other conditions including certain degenerative conditions or structural injury that are not appropriate for this or any exercise and that could result in severe injury if exercise is performed. Accordingly, do not diagnose yourself. See a health professional before you get started. This program makes no warranties express or implied. Exercise at your own risk.

The Lower Back Bible

A Simple Solution to a Pain-Free You

Fred Busch

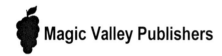 **Magic Valley Publishers**

Published by Magic Valley Publishers
Copyright 2011 © by Fred Busch
All Rights Reserved.

Magic Valley Publishers
6390 E Willow St
Long Beach CA 90815
U.S.A.

ISBN 978-0-9845275-6-4

Cover design by Matt Gonzalez
Manufactured in the United States of America
First Edition

Introduction

Back pain affects millions of men and women. And as the population ages, the situation will continue to worsen. Back pain can be one of the most debilitating types of pain because the spine holds the body together and is involved in almost every movement.

You are probably reading this book because you—or someone you care for—has back pain. You may have tried a number of remedies to eliminate the problem. You may have been told that your back pain is permanent and that you will either have to live with it or undergo surgery.

Before you undertake any course of treatment, you should get the answers to some fundamental, but extremely important questions.

- Why do I have back pain?
- What is the success rate with surgical intervention?
- What are the complications of surgery that might make the pain worse?
- Are there other options?

With the answers to these questions, you will be armed with the information you need to make an informed decision about your course of treatment. I invite you to keep reading, because you need not be resigned to living with pain for the rest of your life.

In this brief book you will learn that back pain is usually not permanent and that back surgery is often not the best solution. You will also learn the most important concept of all:

If you do not address the fundamental source of your back injury, it will probably reoccur regardless of whether surgery or medical intervention alleviates the pain.

Even if your case is extreme and you have lost all hope, there is an excellent chance that the approach outlined in this book will help you to significantly reduce or even eliminate back pain from your life.

This is not a magic cure. It will require effort from you. It will require your attention and commitment. This very specific and carefully sequenced yoga program will become the foundation of your recovery because it addresses the anatomical causes of back pain.

This book is divided into two major sections. Part 1 focuses on individuals suffering from back pain that are new to yoga and its concepts. It discusses anatomy and the typical causes of back pain. It then shows in easy-to-follow illustrated steps the specific yoga poses and sequences you will need to practice. Part II is primarily directed to current yoga practitioners, though in time new students will find it valuable as they gain experience and expertise in their practice. Experienced practitioners will learn how to modify their practice in class to relieve back pain. Additionally, this book will share one of my full power yoga sequences for relieving back pain.

Chapter One — The Healing Environment

A key contributor to relieving or eliminating back pain back pain is creating what is called The Healing Environment. The Healing Environment for the lower back has two major components: doing the things that help improve your strength and balance, and avoiding the things that aggravate or injure you.

First, a warning! While many people come to Yoga for relief from lower back pain, Yoga can make the pain worse almost as easy is it can make it better. This most often happens when a yoga instructor is not masterful in understanding the critical relationship between lower back pain, the hamstrings and forward bends. It is vitally important to make intelligent, careful decisions when employing yoga to heal lower back pain. To fail to do so could make the injury worse.

The good news is that with the simple instructions outlined in this book you can create the perfect Healing Environment where you will never again lift objects with the wrong body alignment or wrong posture; nor will you attempt yoga poses that are going to strain the sacroiliac joint or exacerbate disc problems.

You will, however, learn the specific yoga poses that are going to lengthen your hamstrings without aggravating your lower back in any way.

Chapter Two — My Personal Experience

Some years ago I was practicing a particularly vigorous style of yoga in which heavy adjustments such as pushing on the back during seated-forward-bending are common. As a result, my sacroiliac ligament was overstretched and my sacrum became unstable.[1] The result was lower back pain that typically presented on my left side, but sometimes shifted to my right side. This pain was chronic and seemed like it would never go away. I would have trouble standing and sitting in the car, and practicing yoga had become very painful.

I had never had back pain and it took me some time to realize how pervasive the pain was and how it impacted my ability to function. Since I was always distracted by pain, it was very difficult to live joyfully. I understood how important it was to free myself of this pain. Fortunately, the tools—a combination of yoga and natural healing modalities—were readily available to me.

Already a yoga instructor for many years, with extensive expertise in healing injuries, I turned my attention to my own back pain. After examining the fundamental anatomical causes of back pain and back injury, I developed a Healing Sequence for the Lower Back. This sequence eliminated my back pain, and I have used it successfully on scores of others with differing degrees of pain.

This program can and will help you to live pain free.

---

[1]We will discuss this joint and anatomy in much more detail later. For the moment it is important to understand that an unstable joint is a joint that allows movement is a manner that is abnormal and cannot support normal loads.

Chapter Three — Why Back Pain Is Usually Lower Back Pain

It's estimated that 65 million Americans suffer from lower back pain, the second most common reason for medical visits. It's also estimated that an individual with lower back pain is likely to have one serious episode of back pain every 15 years. Why? The answer can be found in an examination of the fundamental structure of the human body. Humans are unique among mammals in that they are capable of efficient bipedal locomotion. In other words, we can walk and run on two legs.

If you consider the balance and muscular coordination required in the core of your body, you can see that this is an amazing feat. For example, you have well- developed gluteal abductors on the sides of your hips that keep you from falling over in mid-stride. Your thighbone or femur also slopes inward from your hip to the knee thereby keeping your feet under your center of gravity. Apes lack these characteristics and can only walk upright awkwardly for short distances.

Nevertheless, while standing upright is uniquely wonderful, it means that the spine must handle much greater—and entirely different—loads than do the spines of quadrupeds. In a four-legged animal, the pelvis is tilted forward and the spine functions more or less as an anchor for the muscles that support the organs and for body structure. In a human being, the pelvis must be held upright so that the upper body remains balanced over the feet. Figure 3.1. This requires the hamstrings—muscles in the back of the leg—as well as a whole host of other muscles and ligaments to be much tighter and stronger in different ways.

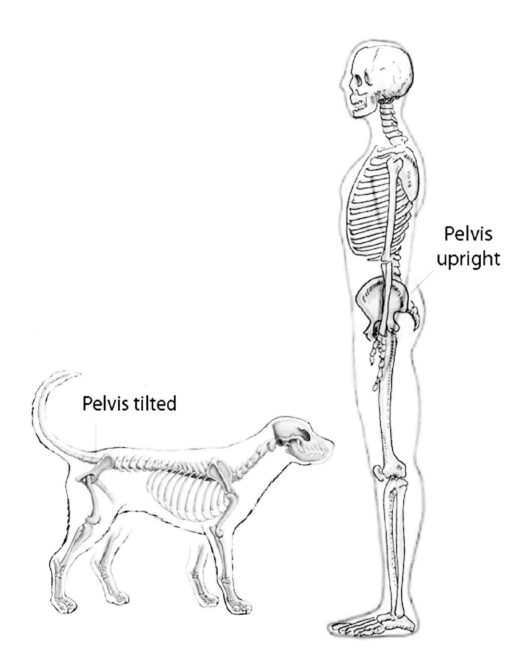

Figure 3.1

What does this have to do with your back pain? The vulnerable link in this chain of muscles, ligaments and tendons that holds you upright is, as you've probably already guessed, the lower back. The relationship between lower back pain and the hamstring muscles will be a key theme throughout this book and will be discussed in greater detail later.

Chapter Four — Common Lower Back Injuries

Let's examine how the lower back is commonly susceptible to injury. In the overwhelming majority of people, lower back pain is caused by one of two distinct conditions: sacroiliac strain and herniated discs of the lumbar vertebrae. We will examine each of these conditions later in detail.

These injuries occur in the lower back rather than the middle or thoracic spine area because there is tremendous range of motion found in the lower back region. And, range of motion means vulnerability to injury.

In contrast, the middle (thoracic) vertebrae are connected and constrained by the rib cage so there is virtually no range of motion in this part of the spine.

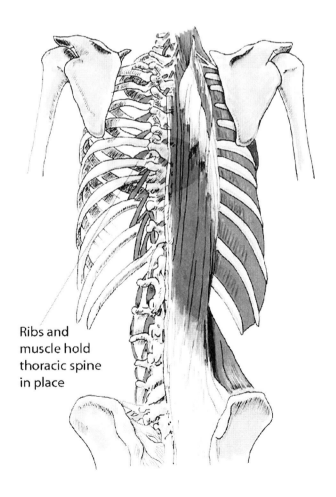

Ribs and muscle hold thoracic spine in place

Figure 4.1.

Thus, the middle back is part of a very rigid structure that includes the ribs and sternum. This is important to remember because any bending that occurs in the back will be concentrated in a relatively small area in the lower back. Figure 4.2. In other words, it is the lower back that takes all the abuse.

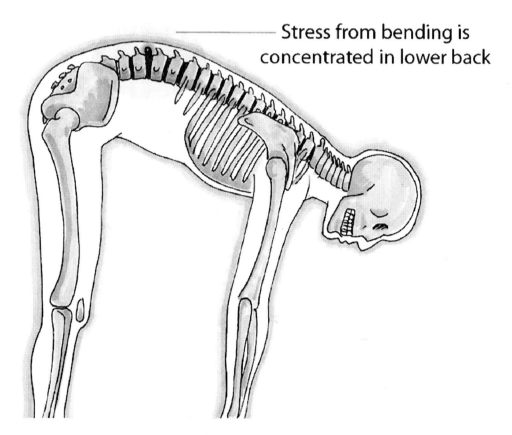

Stress from bending is concentrated in lower back

Figure 4.2

Chapter Five — The Role of the Hamstrings in Lower Back Pain

One of the first things I have students who I train to be yoga instructors memorize is the following relationship: The Hamstrings are attached to the sitting bones. The sitting bones are part of the pelvis. Forward bending requires pelvic rotation. When the hamstrings are tight, pelvic rotation is impeded; and when forward bending occurs, the stress is reflected to the lower back. This can create or exacerbate either sacroiliac strain or herniated discs of the lumbar vertebrae.

You may be wondering at this point why we are only talking about forward bends—not back bends. This is because back bending, when done correctly by engaging the core strength throughout the action, is quite safe.

Now let's take a closer look at the role of the hamstrings in lower back pain. As we discussed briefly above, the relationship between the hamstrings and the inability of the pelvis to tilt forward sufficiently is the key to understanding back pain. Hamstrings are the primary muscle group that restricts the degree of pelvic tilt, which occurs during forward bending. When the pelvis is unable to tilt forward during forward-bending it creates stress in the sacroiliac joint and to the lumbar vertebrae. See Figure 5.1 below.

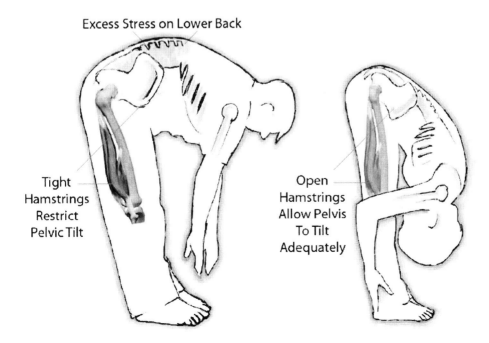

Excess Stress on Lower Back

Tight Hamstrings Restrict Pelvic Tilt

Open Hamstrings Allow Pelvis To Tilt Adequately

Let's locate the hamstrings so that you will be able to visualize where the hamstrings attach to the body. You will then be able to understand why the hamstrings restrict pelvic tilt and cause stress on the back.

The hamstrings are attached to the pelvis. Figure 5.2. The pelvis is actually composed of three different bones: the Ilium, the ischium, and the pubis. The hamstrings are the muscles on the back of your thighs that attach to what is called the ischial tuberosity. The ischial tuberosities are more commonly known as the sitting- bones. You can find your sitting-bones by sitting on the floor and locating the bones that contact the floor.

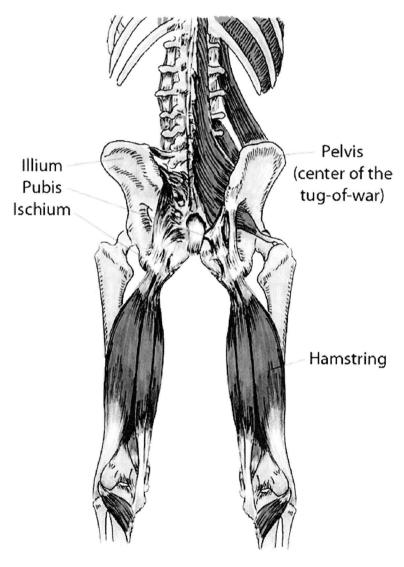

Illium
Pubis
Ischium

Pelvis
(center of the
tug-of-war)

Hamstring

Figure 5.2

The hamstring attachment to the sitting-bones is extremely strong. Because the hamstrings are attached to the very bottom of the pelvis, forward bending can be seen like a tug-of-war between the hamstrings, and the lumbar vertebrae and the sacroiliac joint that are attached on the top of the pelvis. Think of the center point of a tug-of-war rope as the pelvis.

When the hamstrings are too tight (restricting the forward tilt of the pelvis) the rope in the tug of war gets tighter and tighter during forward bending. The weakest point in the rope is the lower back because the hamstrings are stronger than the sacroiliac joint or intervertebral discs. Consequently, the lower back gets injured, not the hamstrings.

Often the injury from forward bending occurs during the simple act of picking up an object from the floor. The stress is increased when the bending is done incorrectly. Instead of bending the knees and keeping the heart lifting (i.e. back flat), most people simply hunch their back and bend at their lower back. When the hamstrings are too tight, pelvic rotation is impeded. Figure 5.3. Forward pelvic rotation cannot occur and the stress then goes directly to the sacroiliac joint and the lumbar vertebrae.

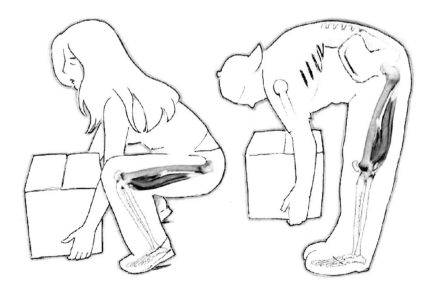

Figure 5.3

To minimize lower back stress, we must lengthen the hamstrings. When the hamstrings do not pull down quite so much, the pelvis is liberated. Even a small degree of lengthening makes a significant difference, and back stress is relieved. Once again, pelvic rotation is essential to pain free movement. The pelvis must be allowed to tilt as much as possible when bending forward. This will reduce the stress in the lower back and allow the back to heal, preventing further injury.

The entire foundation of a pain-free lower back is based upon lengthening the hamstrings in a way that does not implicate the lower back.

Chapter Six — The Movement that Causes Lower Back Pain Is Forward-Bending

Those suffering from lower back pain will often describe the pain as resulting from the act of picking up something heavy. But, more often, the trigger is simple forward bending. The trigger can be something as simple as bending over to brush your teeth.

Forward bending is an integral part of an active live. So, we must pay special attention when we perform a forward bend. Your alignment needs to be perfect to insure that the pelvis is not going to be impeded in the forward-tilting action

It's common advice to bend your knees when picking up heavy objects to reduce potential injury to the back. The reason for this is that during any forward bending, when the pelvis is unable to tilt forward sufficiently, significant stress is created in areas that were not designed to handle this particular kind of load. Those areas are the sacroiliac joint and the discs of the lumbar vertebrae.

To eliminate the risk of causing back pain, we must learn how to correctly forward-bend, how to pick up things from the ground, how to sit and stand. By learning how to forward-bend properly you will eliminate the strain or your lower back. So, in a sense, the prevention and healing of back pain have the same solution, which is proper forward-bending.

Chapter Seven — The Sacroiliac Joint and How It Gets Injured

Before we discuss the sacroiliac joint, it is important to understand a little bit about ligaments, the tough tissue that attaches bones to bones. A slinky is an excellent analogy. Pull it apart and it will return to its natural shape. But, also like a slinky, when the ligament is stretched too far, it will not return to its original shape.

Ligaments and tendons are made from the same material. The difference is that ligaments do not contain blood vessels and are known as avascular. Ligaments must receive nutrients through diffusion from the surrounding joint or tissue. Because they are poorly supplied with nutrients, they are unable to heal quickly relative to the other tissues in your body that do have access a direct supply of nutrients through blood vessels. Thus, when we injure a ligament, recovery is usually very slow … if at all.

Because the sacroiliac joint is one of the most vulnerable areas in the back, we'll now review how this joint is structured and why it is subject to injury. Understanding this will help you to understand how to take care of your sacroiliac and avoid injury.

The sacroiliac joint is located where the sacrum meets the Ilium. Figure 7.1. Most of us have two dimples on our lower back. They mark the location of the sacroiliac joint where the sacrum meets the Ilium. Significantly, it is the only place on the body where the lower extremity bones are attached to the trunk bones. The other attachments of the lower extremity to the upper extremity are through muscular attachment. Thus, the sacroiliac joint is important because it is the only joint that connects your lower extremities (legs and hips) to your spine.

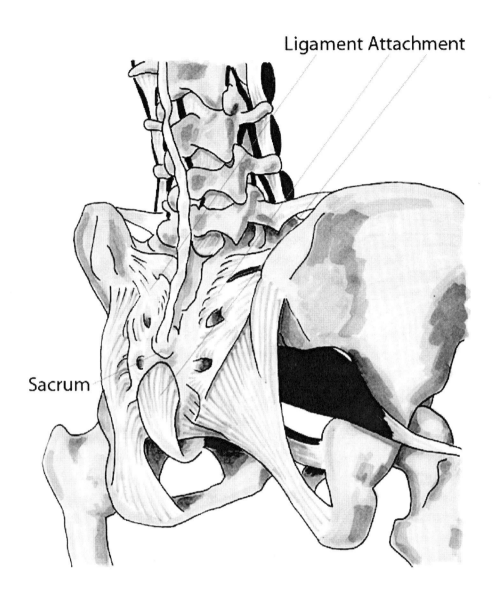

Ligament Attachment

Sacrum

Figure 7.1

Why is this bone-to-bone attachment significant? Because, when sacroiliac joint injury is causing lower back pain, it is a relatively long-term situation. Your goal is to make sure that you do what is necessary to start the healing process and keep it going. You need to relieve the stress on this joint and allow it to heal.

Normally the sacrum is held very tightly into place on the Ilium. Figure 7.1. This joint, when functioning normally, will only allow a small amount of movement called nutation and counter-nutation that is related to the pelvis and the sacrum.

TIP FOR YOGA PRACTITIONERS: While yoga is unquestionably the path to the Divine and incredibly beneficial to the mind and body, asana practiced carelessly can cause serious injury to the lower back. In forward-bend adjustments, where the teacher comes behind the student and pushes the student down in a straight, closed-leg-forward bend, the sacroiliac ligament in highly susceptible to injury. See Figure 7.3. Done correctly (with the heart lifting and emphasis on pelvic tilt) and with the right candidate (someone with relatively open hamstrings) this adjustment can be safe. However, in my experience, 99% of the time these conditions do not exist and this adjustment is unsafe. So, if you have back pain, say "no thanks" to this type of adjustment.

When you have improper forward bending as discussed earlier, the sacroiliac ligament becomes overstretched. The result is a "destabilized sacrum" where the sacroiliac ligaments are lose. A destabilized joint is just a fancy way of saying that the joint can move beyond its normal range of motion.

Because the sacroiliac ligament is overstretched, the sacrum can now pop out of place and be misaligned. This can occur very quickly once the sacroiliac ligament is overstretched because the ligament is not there to do its job. The sacrum becomes out of alignment, either to one side or to the other, up or down or forward and backward. Refer back to figure 7.1 and take a look at the ligaments holding the sacrum in place. If any of these ligaments are loose this flat bone will move in a way in which it was not designed. The immediate result is usually lower back pain. The pain will be significant because once the sacrum is out of place all the muscles in that area must compensate. This compensation causes the muscles to become inflamed and impinge on the nerves.

The important thing to remember here is that the sacroiliac joint can be taken care of properly by lengthening the hamstrings and proper knees-bent, heart-lifting forward-bending. In the coming chapters, we will analyze exactly why the hamstrings, and their relative tightness, play such a critical role in the lower back.

Finally, the sacroiliac joint will heal, but that healing process can take much longer than we would like.

Luckily, we don't mind how long the sacroiliac joint takes to heal because this program will relieve pain now.

A FEW WORDS ABOUT HAVING YOUR SACRUM CHECKED: Once the sacrum is destabilized, it has the tendency to shift, the result of any number of activities that you engage in during your daily life. An occasional visit to a holistic chiropractor can be very helpful in speeding the healing process because he or she can make bone adjustments almost impossible to do by yourself. Select a chiropractor that understands other healing modalities and uses chiropractic mastery in conjunction with proper exercise and stretching.

Chapter Eight — Herniated Discs

The other common condition that leads to back pain is a herniated disc. In this chapter we will discuss what a herniated disc is, how this type of herniation occurs, how it causes pain, and how you can alleviate this pain.

The word hernia means protrusion or rupture. A hernia is a rupture through the fascia layer that is supposed to contain that tissue. For example, a common herniation occurs in the inner groin where the connection between muscles rips and allows organs to slightly protrude.

In the case of the spine, a much smaller but potentially painful herniation can occur. The main structure of the spine consists of vertebrae (bones) and discs. See Figure 8.1. The intervertebral discs are made of cartilage, the same material in the nose and ears and a variety of other connective tissues. The discs are designed to act as shock absorbers in the vertebrae and to connect each vertebra to the one above and below. They are encased in a protective sheath.

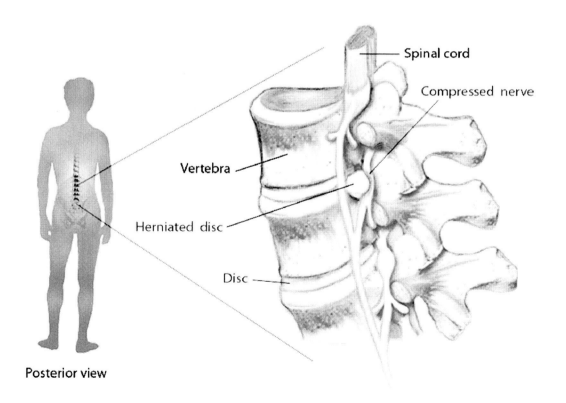

Spinal cord

Compressed nerve

Vertebra

Herniated disc

Disc

Posterior view

Figure 8.1

When you incorrectly forward-bend, or subject your back to other trauma, the inside of the disc itself can rupture through the sheath or covering. Forward bending has a strong tendency to cause this injury, especially when combined with a twist. Sometimes the disc does not fully rupture, but bulges out. This is known as a bulging disc. A bulging disc can be painful in the same way as a herniated disc.

These disc problems are significant because the spine is the main nerve pathway through the body. When the intervertebral disc ruptures, it has the potential to impinge or affect a nerve and cause pain. In addition, the herniated discs will also create a compensational mechanism where the muscles in the back tighten to protect the injured area. This, of course, can also result in severe pain. Symptoms of a herniated disc are often tingling or shooting pain in the back or extremities, abnormal muscle tightness and spasms in the back.

Having said this, we should **not** make herniated discs into more than they are because they are very common. In fact, many people have a herniated disc and they are not even aware of it. In rare cases, these people may go their entire life and never be aware that they have a herniated disc because it doesn't impinge the nerve and it doesn't create pain.

Herniated discs will not heal on their own however; we don't need them to heal to live pain free.

We want to avoid things that would make the herniation worse and we want to relieve the stress and pain from that area. So, first, no forward bending! Forward bending is going to put pressure on the disk to herniate or bulge further. Second, we want to strengthen the surrounding core muscles to support this area as much as possible.

Simple, daily exercise regimens (yoga sequencing) will help you maintain a properly structured, healthy, pain-free body.

Chapter Nine — Best Exercise for Lower Back Pain

One of the most common questions a yoga instructor is asked is "what is the best yoga pose to heal my back pain?" Unfortunately, it's not as simple as doing a single exercise. As we discussed earlier, the lower back is at the core of the body: muscles, bones, ligaments and tendons all connect, coordinating and communicating with each other. Accordingly, a comprehensive sequence of exercises is required to address this highly complex physical system.

Certainly, one important goal is to lengthen the hamstrings, but stretching the hamstrings alone is not enough. The hamstrings must be lengthened in the context of the rest of the body getting stronger, healthier and more flexible as well.

Your focus will be on opening the hamstrings and strengthening other key areas of your body to support lower back health. In addition, you will avoid movements and exercises that cause or aggravate your pain.

The intelligent, conscious, integration of the body that results from intelligent exercise (yoga poses) and awareness will lead to a dramatically improved quality of life.

Chapter Ten — A Word of Caution

Now, let's discuss the specific poses needed for the healing sequences.

But first a word of caution.

- Poses done incorrectly have the potential to make your situation worse.
- Poses are intended to be performed in sequence and in a certain manner.
- Pease read this section through to the end, and only then perform the poses in the sequences described.

Chapter Eleven — The Healing Sequence Key Yoga Poses Explored Individually

This chapter introduces each of the key yoga poses in the healing sequence. Pay close attention to the detailed description of each pose, even if you are an experienced yoga practitioner. Perform the poses only in the sequences described later in this book.

Downward Dog

Downward Dog is perhaps the most widely recognized yoga pose. It is an important pose with numerous benefits because it strengthens the upper body and core while providing a mild stretch to the back of the legs. Downward Dog is generally safe and beneficial for the back when performed properly.

Figure 11.1 is an illustration of a classical Downward Dog. However, if you have lower back pain there is a good chance that you have tight hamstrings, which will impede the tilt of your pelvis, and your Downward Dog may look like Figure 11.2. This puts strain on your lower back for all the reasons we discussed in the preceding chapters. The solution is to bend your knees. Figure 11.3 illustrates the correct adjustment of Downward Dog for a person with tight hamstrings.

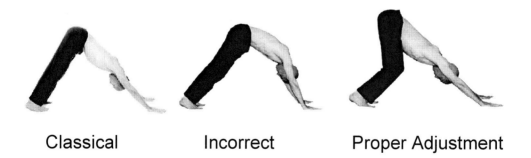

Classical   Incorrect   Proper Adjustment

Cobra

Cobra pose is illustrated below. As you can see, cobra pose is a back bend.

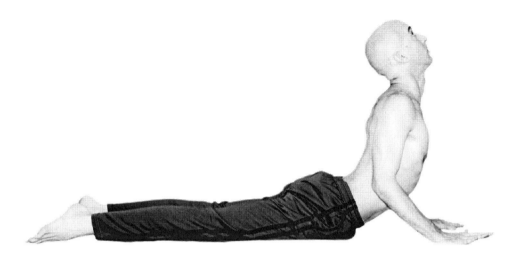

There are three essential rules to follow when back-bending.

- First, be gentle. Do not try to bend too high. A gentle bend performed properly will be much safer and more beneficial.
- Second, protect your lower back from excess compression by rotating your pelvis properly. Note that by rotating your pelvis away from the bend (drawing your navel towards your spine) you are preventing an excess compression stress on your lower back.
- Third, expand the front of your body to make a larger arch. This will also prevent excess compression of your spine. While it is not obvious to most people, back bending is really all about stretching your front.

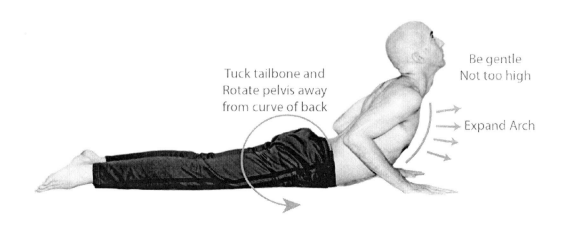

Tuck tailbone and
Rotate pelvis away
from curve of back

Be gentle
Not too high

Expand Arch

Plank

Plank pose is excellent for strengthening the core and results in much-needed muscular support for the back. Slightly elevate the buttocks and hold the legs and abdomen and back tight.

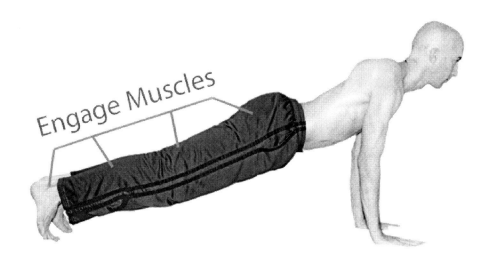

Engage Muscles

Do not let the back sag. If your wrists are sensitive to the pressure of this pose, it may be performed on the forearms.

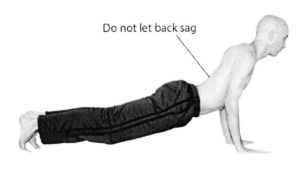

Do not let back sag

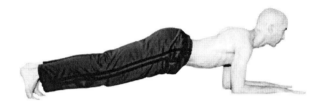

To perform a yoga push-up, hands should be about shoulder-width apart. Lower down and rise up slowly with elbows next to the body.

Warrior 1

For Warrior 1 pose the front knee is bent but not beyond the toes. Both feet should be flat and firm on the ground. Upper body and hips should face squarely forward. As you look up, perform a mild back-bend. The same principles that we discussed regarding Cobra pose apply here. Be gentle, expand your front body and work the pelvis to tilt against the back-bend to prevent excess compression. Also make sure that your chest is lifting up to the ceiling.

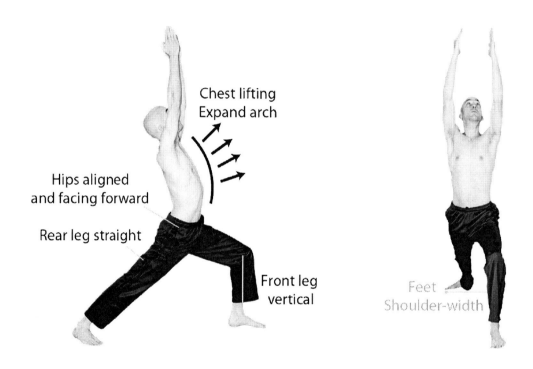

Warrior 2

In Warrior 2 pose, your feet are aligned and your stance is a bit wider. See Below. Rather that squaring the hips forward as in Warrior 1, you should open the hips in line with the feet. Attempt to rotate the pelvis back to obtain more opening of the hips.

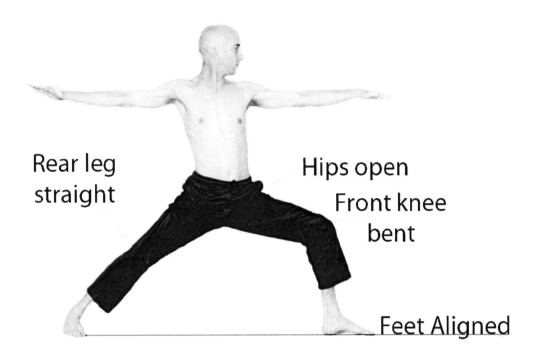

Rear leg straight

Hips open
Front knee bent

Feet Aligned

Side-Angle

In Side-Angle pose, the lower body is in essentially the same position as Warrior 2. Those with back pain should perform this pose with the elbow on the thigh. And then reach over your head. Keep the spine as straight as possible.

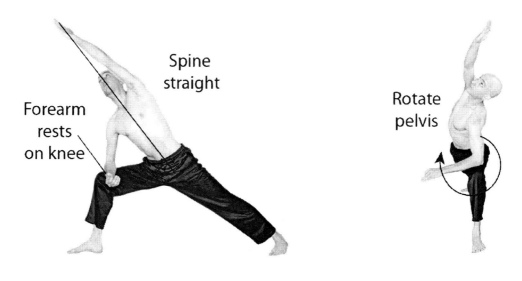

Warrior 3

Warrior 3 is one of the more formidable yoga poses, even for an experienced practitioner; however, it is relatively safe and beneficial when performed to any degree that you can. Begin in Warrior 1 and place hands on hips. Lean forward as you raise your rear leg. If this is easy for you, reach your arms straight out. This pose can also be performed with hands against the wall or on a chair.

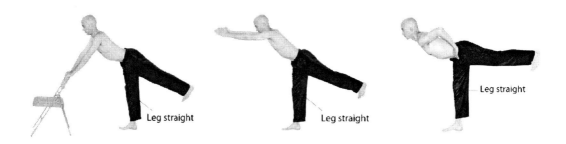

Pull On Straight Leg

This is the single most important pose.

Lay flat on your back. Use a strap, towel, or something similar to lasso your foot. There are two things that you absolutely must do during this pose.

- First, keep your opposite leg engaged and firmly on the ground. This will help keep your pelvis in a neutral position on the ground. To do this simply arch your lower back slightly off the ground and set it down. Notice the direction that your pelvis rotated. Don't allow it to rotate the other way.
- Second, keep your raised leg perfectly straight.

Now pull gently on your straight leg to safely open your hamstrings. It's ok if you feel mild pain in your hamstrings as long as you are being gentle.

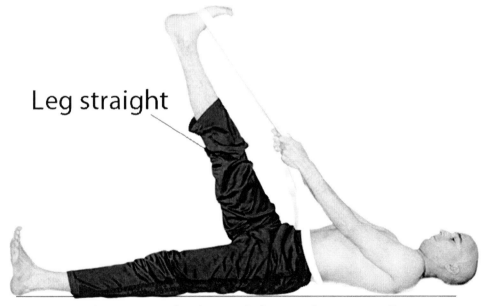

Leg straight

Pelvis and shoulders flat on floor

Chapter Twelve — Why the Straight-Leg, One-Legged Pull Is Important

As discussed earlier, the hamstrings often restrict pelvic rotation. We also discussed the importance of lengthening the hamstrings to reduce the pressure on the other side of the pelvic attachment of the sacroiliac joint. Therefore, we need ways to lengthen the hamstrings without stressing the back.

The safest, simplest and most effective way I have found is the Supta Padangustasana pose. In plain English, lie on your back and pull on one straight leg at a time with a belt or strap. For this to be effective, you must keep your leg straight. Most likely you will need a strap if your hamstrings are at all tight. Most people, when they attempt this pose, put a slight bend to the knee. It's really important, however, that you feel that your leg is locked. There should be no bending, not even a "micro-bend," in the knee.

Some yoga poses require significant bending in the knee. This is not one of them. Allowing the knee to bend, even slightly, will bring the stress into the tendon and not the hamstring muscle.

TIP: *As you pull on your straight leg, engage (tighten) your quadriceps (front of your leg). Your body will automatically relax the hamstring. This is called reciprocal inhibition.*

Create a straight, locked, and muscularly-engaged leg with arms straight as well. Why is this simple pose so effective? Because it allows you to stretch your hamstrings and keep your lower back in a safe position. When you lie on your back and keep your opposite leg on the floor, your hips are aligned with the floor and your back is kept from bending like in a forward-bend. See above.

Look again at Warrior 3 pose and you will see that it is very similar with a different orientation. Of course, Warrior 3 is much more challenging because you must hold your leg up. Because of the similar anatomical benefit, Warrior

3—with your hands on the wall—is also one of the most important healing poses for the lower back.

But, the straight-legged one-legged pull is the center of it all. Accessing the hamstring directly this way provides length to the hamstring, which will reduce the tension on the ischial tuberosity and reduce the pull downward on the sitting bones and the stress on the sacroiliac ligament or the herniated disc.

The straight-legged one-legged pull must be done every single day without exception.

Chapter Thirteen — Assessing your Back Pain

Now let's focus on the different areas of the body where back pain is experienced and how they relate to identifying the source of the pain. The critical question is: Where is the exact location of the pain that you are feeling? Is it at the lowest part of your back, closer to your buttocks? This kind of pain correlates to what we referred to earlier as the sacroiliac joint. Figure 13.1. Pain in the sacroiliac joint may exhibit the following symptoms:

- It comes and goes,

- It moves from one side to the other,

- It can never really be massaged to relief, and

- Sensations can either be dull and annoying-to-sharp and startling.

Or, is your pain in the spine, rather than the sacrum? Pain higher up in the spine, but still in the lower back is often a sign of potential herniated discs. Pain in the lower spine can shoot down the leg via the sciatic nerve. Basically, if you have lower back pain and the pain is not located in the sacral region, it is then related to the lumbar vertebrae, and the muscles and nerves connecting and innervating the lumbar.

The final option for the source of back pain could involve the cervical vertebrae, but that would be more commonly known as 'neck pain' and might be the result of whiplash or other causes. This book will not cover the subject of neck pain, but the basic rules are not to turn your head if it hurts and NEVER do a headstand or shoulder stand unless you are with a yoga master who has practiced and taught for at least 20 years, and even then it may be questionable.

The sequences we will be doing are equally safe and effective for both pain originating in the sacroiliac joint and in the lumbar discs. Nevertheless, it is important that you identify the difference if possible. If you have a disc injury, you need to be much more careful with any type of twisting. Mild twisting movements than occur during everyday activities can aggravate and often severely worsen disc injuries, especially when the twist is combined with a forward bend.   So, if you have a disc injury please be mindful of avoiding asymmetrical unconscious twisting movements.

It is always wise prior to beginning any exercise program to consult a physician. This is particularly true in the case of back pain because the extent of your injury may not correlate with the pain you are experiencing.

Chapter Fourteen — Putting it all Together: Specific Sequences for Healing Back Pain

We have now arrived at the yoga sequences that will, over time, help you reduce and hopefully eliminate your back pain. The following are three complete yoga sequences of progressive intensity. Begin with "Sequence I for Healing Back Pain." Once you are comfortable with that sequence and your back pain begins to recede, you may then move onto the more rigorous "Sequence II for Healing Back Pain" and then to the "Sequence III for Healing Back Pain" when you are pain free.

Progress slowly; starting with the initial sequence because the amount of pain you are experiencing may not correlate with the severity of the injury to your back. Some people experience a high degree of pain with a relatively mild injury and others experience minimal pain with a more serious injury. The sequences are designed to allow you to progress and build both strength and critical flexibility.

Please review Chapter 11 before beginning and while performing each pose. Performing these poses correctly is critical for obtaining the desired results. Please try not to evaluate how "well" you are doing; just follow the instructions specifically and don't worry about how strong or flexible you are.

You will need a yoga mat and a strap. A number of household items such as an old belt will do fine.

If possible, find or create a warm environment in which to practice. If that is not possible, take a warm bath or shower before you begin.

SEQUENCE I – Initial Practice

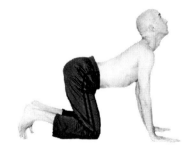

Cow Pose – Inhale

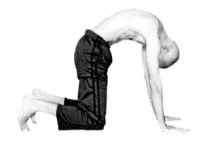

Cat Pose - Exhale

----- Repeat 4 more times -----

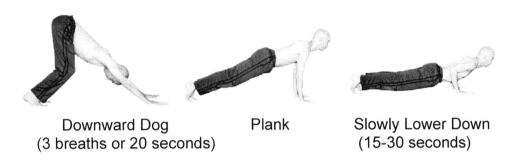

| Downward Dog | Plank | Slowly Lower Down |
| (3 breaths or 20 seconds) | | (15-30 seconds) |

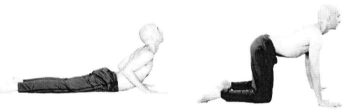

| Cobra | Hands and Knees |
| (up and down 3 times) | (1 Breath or more) |

----- Repeat 2 more times -----

Stand carefully as follows:

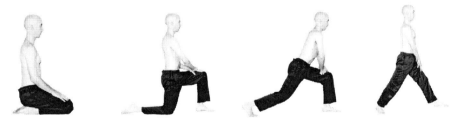

Step one foot forward so the foot is directly under its knee and place your hands on your thigh. Then extend your bent knee as you push your arms into your leg and stand up. Your spine should be straight and close to vertical the entire time.

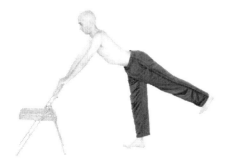 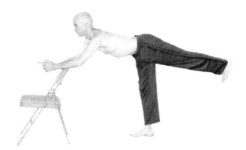

Warrior 3 with Chair
(Beginner)

Warrior 3 with Chair
(Advanced beginner option)

Perform Warrior 3 on left and right side (3 breaths or 20 seconds)

----- Repeat -----

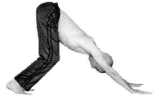 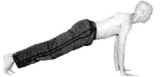 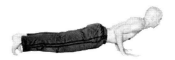

Downward Dog
(3 breaths or 20 seconds)

Plank

Slowly Lower Down
(15-30 seconds)

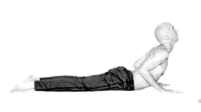 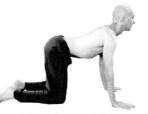

Cobra
(up and down 3 times)

Hands and Knees
(1 Breath or more)

----- Repeat 2 more times -----

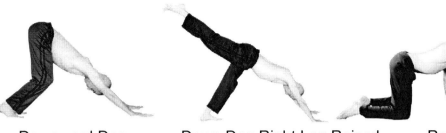

Downward Dog
(1 Breath)

Down Dog Right Leg Raised
(5 breaths or 30 seconds)

Rest

----- Repeat sequence with left leg raised -----

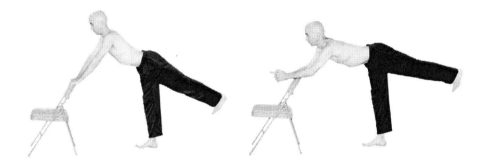

Warrior 3 with Chair
(Beginner)

Warrior 3 with Chair
(Advanced beginner option)

Perform Warrior 3 on left and right side (3 breaths or 20 seconds)

----- Repeat 2 more times -----

Stand carefully as instructed above

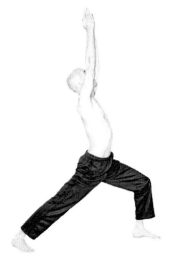 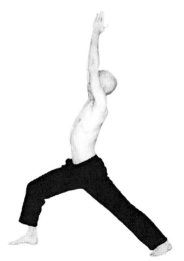

Warrior 1 - Left Side
(3 Breaths or 20 Seconds)

Warrior 1 – Right Side
(3 Breaths or 20 Seconds)

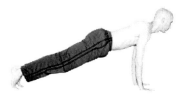 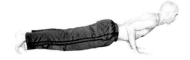

OPTIONAL- Push ups or push ups on knees.
(as many as you can do under control)

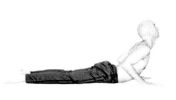 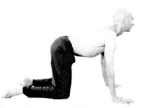 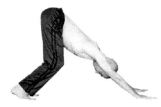

Cobra
(up and down 3 times)

Hands and Knees
(1 Breath or more)

Downward Dog
(5 Breaths or 30 seconds)

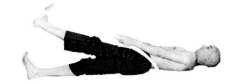 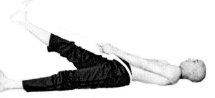

Pull on straight leg with strap–Left
(30 Seconds or 5 Breaths)

Pull on straight leg with strap–Right
(30 Seconds of 5 Breaths)

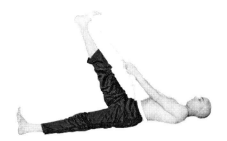

Advanced Position Option
(for students with more hamstring flexibility)

--- Repeat 3 times each side ---

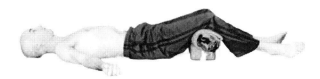

Savasana - final rest with bolster or blankets under the knees.

Five minutes or longer

SEQUENCE II

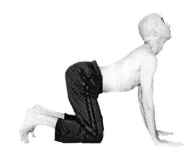 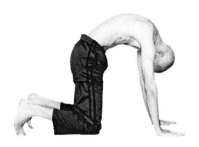

Cow Pose – Inhale   Cat Pose - Exhale

----- Repeat 4 more times -----

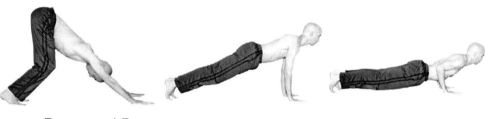

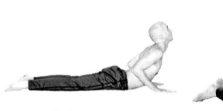

Downward Dog
(3 breaths or 20 seconds)

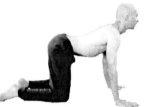

Push Ups (5 – 10 repetitions)

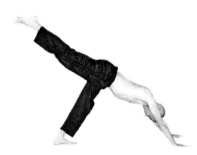

Cobra
(up and down 3 times)

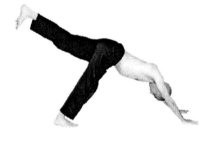

Hands and Knees
(1 Breath or more)

----- Repeat 2 more times -----

Three Leg Dog on Left
(5 Breaths or 30 Seconds)

Three Leg Dog on Right
(5 Breaths or 30 Seconds)

----- Rest 1 Breath and Repeat -----

Stand carefully as follows

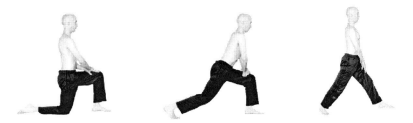

Step one foot forward so the foot is directly under its knee and place your hands on your thigh. Then extend your bent knee as you push your arms into your leg and stand up. Your spine should be straight and close to vertical the entire time.

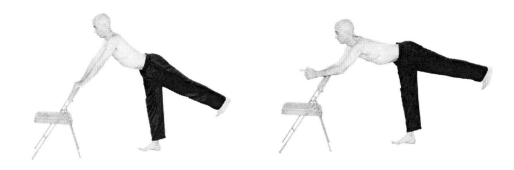

Warrior 3 with Chair
(Beginner)

Warrior 3 with Chair
(Advanced beginner option)

Perform Warrior 3 on left and right side (5 breaths or 30 seconds)

----- Repeat 2 more times -----

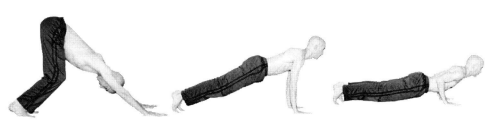

Downward Dog
(3 breaths or 20 seconds)

Push Ups (5 – 10 repetitions)

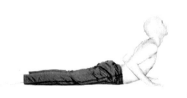 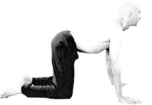

Cobra	Hands and Knees
(up and down 3 times)	(1 Breath or more)

----- Repeat 2 more times -----

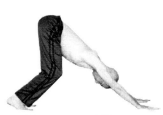 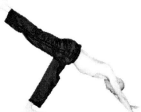 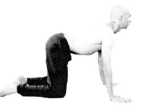

Downward Dog	Down Dog Right Leg Raised	Rest
(1 Breath)	(5 breaths or 30 seconds)	

----- Repeat sequence with left leg raised -----
---Repeat entire sequence both sides---

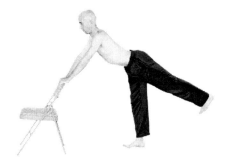 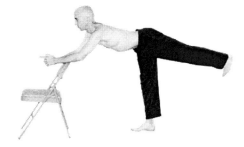

Warrior 3 with Chair	Warrior 3 with Chair
(Beginner)	(Advanced beginner option)

Perform Warrior 3 on left and right side (3 breaths or 20 seconds)

----- Repeat 2 more times -----

Stand carefully as instructed above

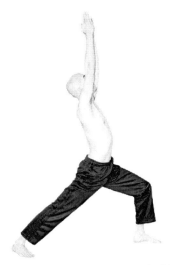 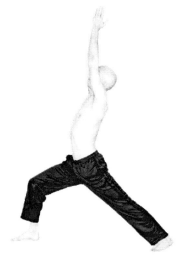

Warrior 1 - Left Side	Warrior 1 – Right Side
(3 Breaths or 20 Seconds)	(3 Breaths or 20 Seconds)

----Repeat 3 times----

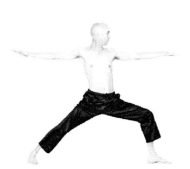 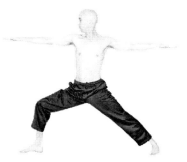

Warrior 2 - Left Side	Warrior 2 – Right Side
(3 Breaths or 20 Seconds)	(3 Breaths or 20 Seconds)

----Repeat 3 times----

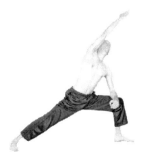 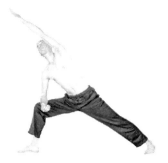

Side Angle - Left Side
(3 Breaths or 20 Seconds)

Side Angle – Right Side
(3 Breaths or 20 Seconds)

----Repeat 2 times----

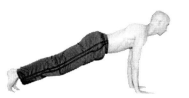 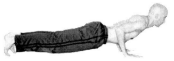

OPTIONAL- Push ups or push ups on knees.
(as many as you can do under control)

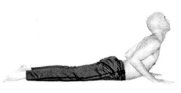 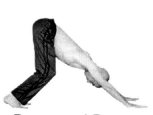

Cobra   Hands and Knees   Downward Dog
(up and down 3 times) (1 Breath or more) (5 Breaths or 30 seconds)

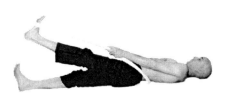 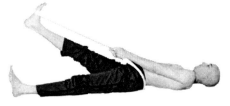

Pull on straight leg with strap-Left   Pull on straight leg with strap-Right
(30 Seconds or 5 Breaths)   (30 Seconds of 5 Breaths)

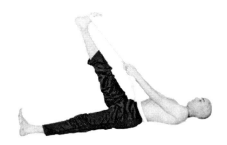

Advanced Position Option
(for students with more hamstring flexibility)

--- Repeat 3 times each side ---

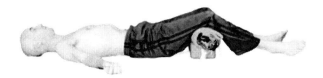

Savasana - final rest with bolster or blankets under the knees.

Five minutes or longer

Once you are comfortable with Sequence II you may advance to the full power yoga sequence in Chapter 24.

Chapter Fifteen — Review

Let's review the key points:

- Forward-bending is the usual source of low back pain and injury because the hamstrings are stronger than both the sacroiliac joint and the lumbar intervertebral discs, so all of the stress of bending goes into the back.

- To prevent further injury try to avoid forward-bending unless the knees are significantly bent.

- Lengthen the hamstrings to reduce stress on the lower back and strengthen core muscles to provide support to the injured area.

- Hamstring lengthening and core strengthening can be accomplished safely by following the sequences outlined above.

The rest is up to you. Let go of the past and realize that you can live pain free.

Guidance for Yoga Practitioners

The following chapters are directed to yoga practitioners with lower back pain. They will show you how to practice in a way that will help alleviate your pain. Let me assure you that some basic modifications of your practice will make an immediate and dramatic difference.

Perhaps you began practicing yoga to ease your existing back pain or you are an avid yogi who has nagging back pain resulting from asana practice or some other source. Whatever the reason, the solution has the same three components:

- Avoid injurious poses,
- Perform beneficial poses, and
- Strengthen key areas for core muscular support.

Note: I am assuming that you have relatively moderate-to-mild back pain and that you currently practice yoga. If you have moderate-to-severe pain, begin with the healing sequences in Part I of this book until your pain is relieved…only then should you return to your regular practice.

Chapter Sixteen — Anatomy of Back Pain

From the preceding chapters you know that the key to alleviating back pain is lengthening the hamstrings without stressing the lower back. This is accomplished by controlling the tilt of the pelvis. We will cover all of the common poses and how to properly perform them and you will learn how to modify and tailor your practice to your specific needs.

Chapter Seventeen — Presence and Mindfulness

Even those who regularly practice yoga can from time to time forget that the physical exercise is only one aspect of the discipline. While this is not intended to be a book about the philosophical aspects of yoga, I'd like to take a moment to reinforce several fundamental ideas in the context of what we are doing to relieve your back pain.

Presence and **Mindfulness**

You may have been exposed to these concepts depending upon the type of instruction you have received. The basic idea of Presence is that the path to true enlightenment and bliss comes through being focused on the present moment rather than events of the past or worry about the future. Similarly, Mindfulness in a broad sense refers to being cognizant of how your actions affect yourself and others.

What does this have to do your back pain? What you do in any particular yoga session should not be influenced in any way by:

- What other people in the class are doing,
- What you have been able to do in the past,
- What you anticipate doing in the future, or
- Your ego.

You must be in the present moment. You must understand what is beneficial for you in that moment and be mindful that you are doing yourself no harm.

Yoga is not a sport or a competition. It's a personal experience. There are beneficial ways to perform poses (depending on your individual anatomy), but there is no "right" way and "wrong" way. Being "good" at yoga has nothing to do with whether you can touch your toes or put your leg behind your head. In simple terms, the goal is to perform each pose in a way that is most beneficial to you. If you can do that, then your practice is perfect, regardless of the physical appearance of the posture.

Be mindful of what you are doing. Don't let your ego drive you to overstretch or perform poses that are going to injure you.

Chapter Eighteen — What to do in Yoga Class

Hopefully, you have a yoga class that you enjoy. How can you incorporate the concepts in this book into that class? First, free your mind of the idea that you must do whatever the instructor calls out. As we discussed above, yoga is a completely personal experience. It's not a military boot camp. You must modify your practice in a way that is beneficial to you, based on the specific poses we will discuss. Every experienced yoga instructor understands this concept. If you sense otherwise, find another instructor.

Now a brief word about adjustments. Different yoga styles have different approaches to adjustment of students' poses. Adjustments range from no adjustment to gentle touch to aggressive physical alignment. All of these approaches are valid so long as they are performed by an experienced instructor. Certainly the aggressive physical alignment approach has the highest potential to cause injury. The best approach is to inform your instructor before class that you have a history of lower back pain. And never be shy about saying "no thank you" to a particular adjustment.

Finally, some styles of yoga involve a lot of aggressive forward-bending. You can—and should—modify any sequence in a way that is intelligent for your back; however, it might be easier to simply find a style that is more conducive to what you are trying to accomplish.

Chapter Nineteen — The Warm-Up

Proper warm-up is essential to the safe practice of yoga. Warming up directs blood flow and heat to critical muscles and connective tissue. This will minimize the possibility of injury. It also feels great! Whether practicing at home or in class, perform the following sequence at the start of your practice. Please refer to Chapter 11 so that you know how to perform each pose in a way that will not injure your back. Generally, you always want to keep your knees bent in any forward-bending, move slowly and move gently.

NOTE: Yoga instructors tend to be flexible people with very open hamstrings and no back pain. For this reason less experienced instructors are sometimes not aware of how their sequences are affecting people who do have back pain and tight hamstrings. It is not uncommon for a yoga class to begin with extensive forward-bending. This is not a good situation for your back pain. We will show you how to modify these bends. Arrive early for class and perform this warm-up sequence.

The following warm-up sequence is shown in detail with photos in Chapter 24 as the opening of my full healing sequence.

Warm-Up Sequence

Alternate Cat and Cow 10x -1 Breath each

Downward Dog with knees bent -5 Breaths

Hands and Knees 1 Breath

Downward Dog with knees bent -5 Breaths

Hands and Knees 1 Breath

Downward Dog with one leg raised -5 Breaths each side

Hands and Knees 1 Breath

Downward Dog/plank/push up/Downward dog -3x

Cobra -3x

Downward Dog with Knees bent

Sun Salutation sequence A (with knees bent) 3x

Sun Salutation sequence B (with knees bent) 3x

Downward Dog right leg knee to nose -5x

Warrior I – 5 breaths

Lunging Warrior – 5 breaths

Bottom of push-up/Upward dog/downward dog

Repeat for left side

Bottom of push-up/upward dog/downward dog

Very good, you should be sweating a little and fairly warm. We are now ready to discuss modifications and beneficial poses.

Chapter Twenty — Modifications and Substitutions

Now let's focus on the common poses that have the potential to injure or aggravate your lower back and discuss ways to modify these poses to make them more beneficial for you.

As you have already surmised from earlier chapters, any pose that involves forward-bending with your legs straight and either together or hip's-width apart has the greatest potential for injury. These poses can have a number of orientations and variations. I will try to cover all of the common poses; but if you encounter something not covered that you suspect may be injurious, it is best to exercise restraint and substitute a pose that you know to be safe for you.

As you perform these poses remember that all the stress goes into your lower back when the hamstrings restrict the tilt of your pelvis when you bend forward. So, you will have a few basic strategies (depending on the pose) for dealing with this situation. Sometimes, you will bend your knees to release the tension from the hamstrings and/or keep your back flat and only bend to the limit of pelvic tilt. The best strategy, however, always is to substitute a pose where the pelvis is held in a safe position. This will become clearer from the illustrations and discussion below.

Standing Bends

Standing bends have a great potential to injure or aggravate your back. The only exception is wide-legged forward bends, which often are fine because the width of the legs allows the pelvis to rotate freely and this is anatomically very different from other standing forward-bends. Either way, you must be very careful when forward-bending in any manner.

Forward Bending

The key in forward-bending is to:

- Bend your knees,
- Stop bending when your pelvis can no longer rotate forward.

When you do this, your back will remain flat and protected from injury. Do not push yourself in this pose, which is a simple way to transition into other poses and warm up. NOT AN INTENSE STRETCH.

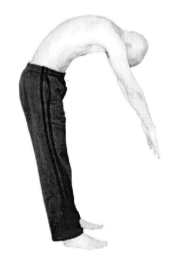   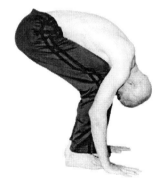

Incorrect   **Correct- Back Safe**

Forward Bend

Pyramid

The key to this pose is to stop bending when your pelvis stops rotating. This means that your back will remain PERFECTLY FLAT. Use blocks as shown in the illustration:

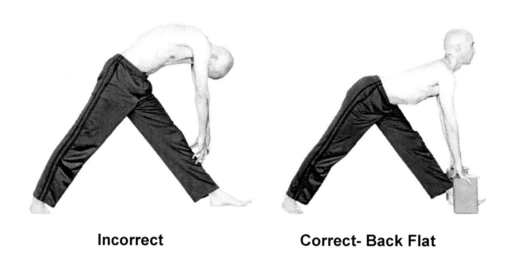

Incorrect   **Correct- Back Flat**

Twisting Triangle

Avoid this pose until you are free of back pain. Substitute gentle Pyramid or Warrior III.

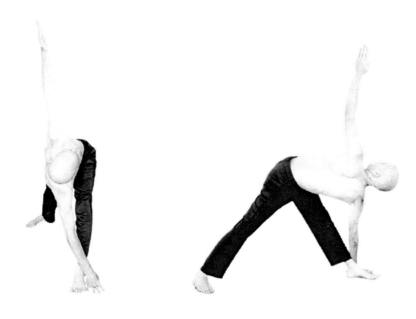

Wide Leg Forward Bend

Avoid this pose if you have significant back pain. If you only have mild pain, you may perform this pose gently with your knees bent and your heart lifting.

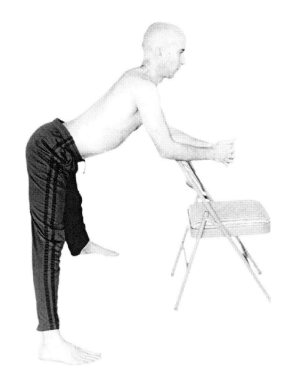

Twisting Half Moon
Avoid this pose. Do Warrior III instead.

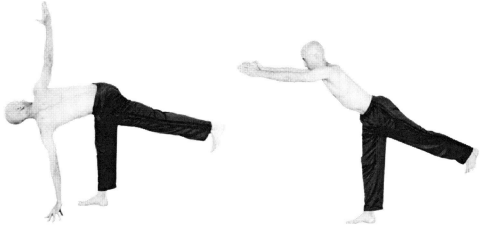

Avoid   Substitute –Warrior III

Balancing Poses

You may perform these poses with the exception of any pose where you would be pulling on your straight leg while standing. You must also keep your back flat/ heart lifting so that your pelvis remains in a safe position for your back.

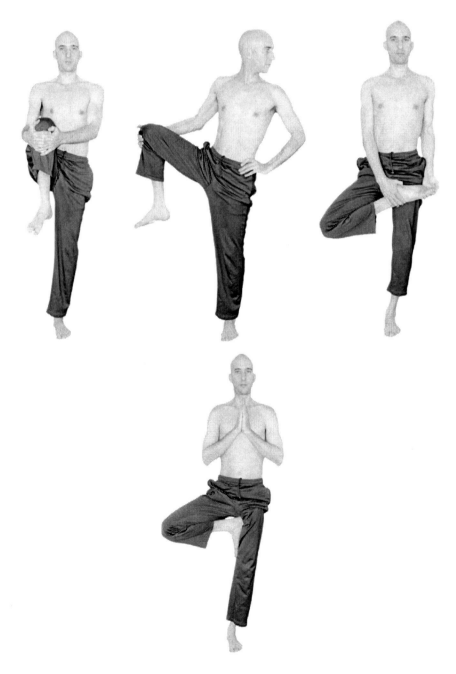

Safe Standing Poses

54

Fred Busch

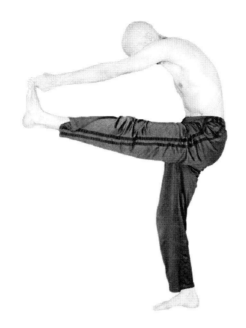

Avoid Straight Leg Standing Poses

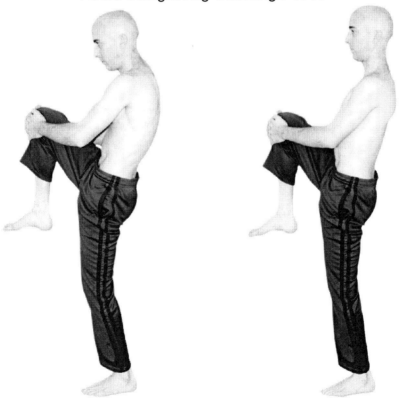

Incorrect   Correct

Keep Back Flat

Twisting Chair

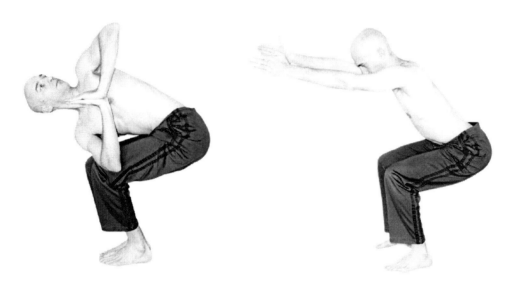

Avoid Twisting Chair Pose   Substitute Chair Pose

Squatting Poses

There are a number of squatting poses and hip-opening poses that are all similar. (Illustration of squatting, elbows down, etc). Avoid these poses; instead perform Downward Dog with knees bent.

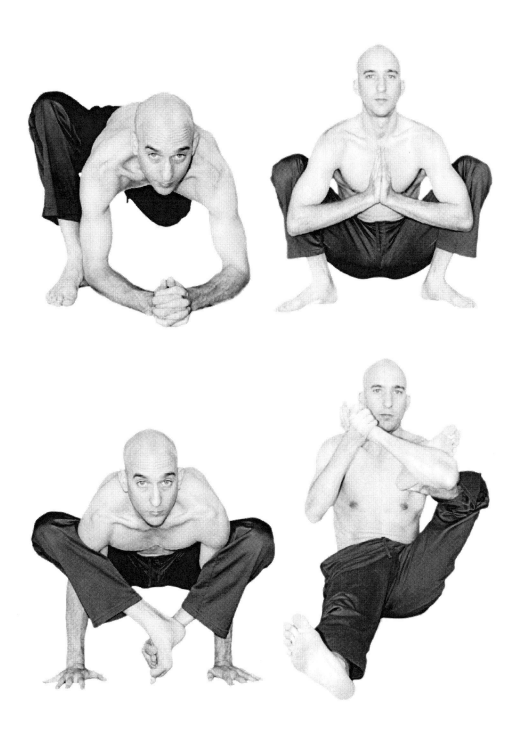

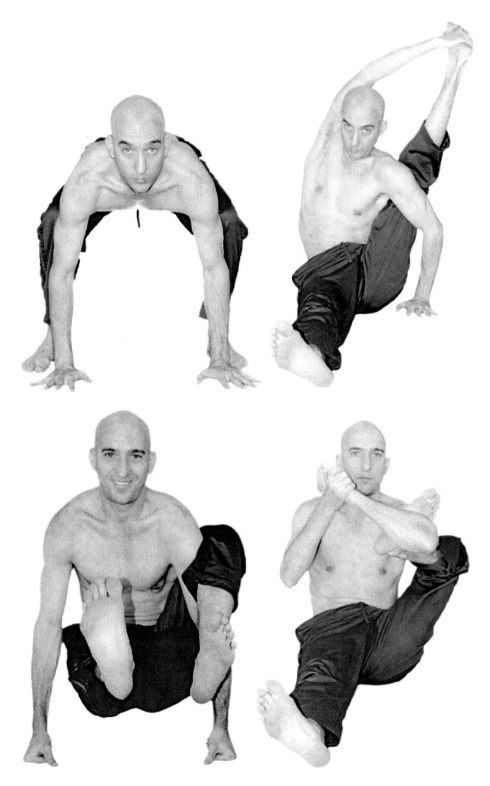

Avoid the Poses Shown Above

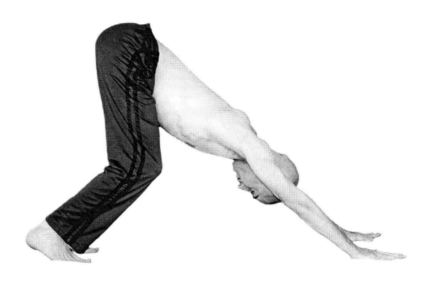

Substitute – Down Dog with Knees Bent

Seated Bends

There are a variety of seated-forward bends. (See illustrations of common seated-forward bends below.) These ARE NOT SAFE for your back. You should substitute lying on your back with a straight leg and strap.

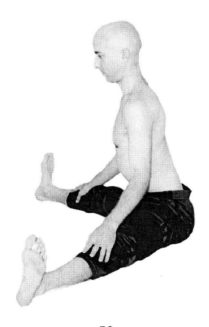

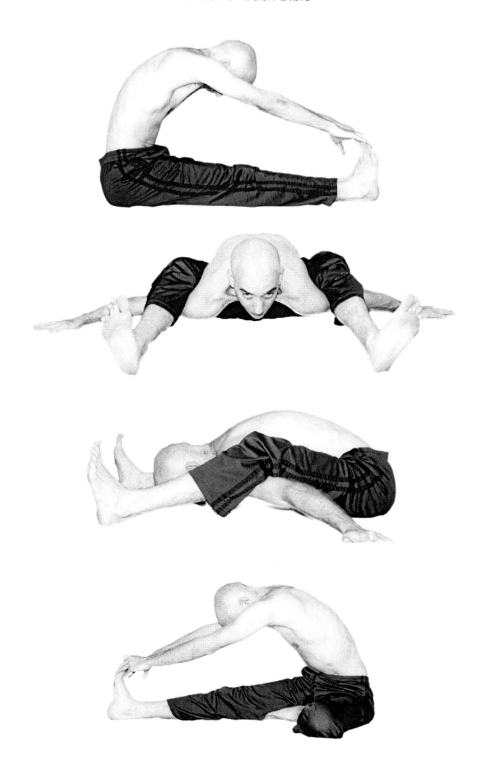

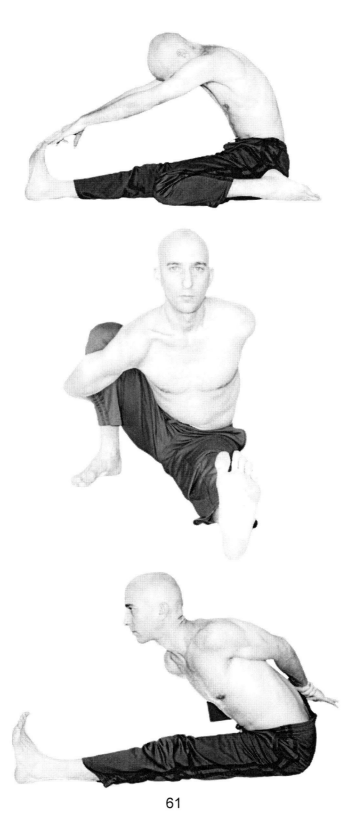

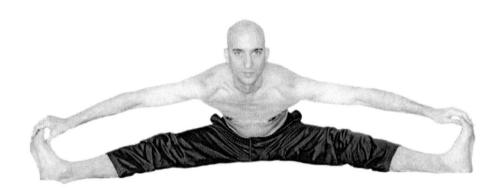

Avoid these poses

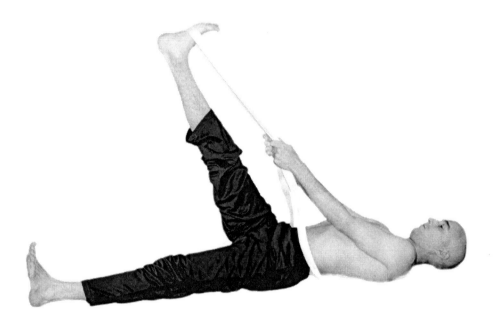

Substitute this Pose

Cobbler

Cobbler is good without the forward-bending aspect. Simply work on bringing the knees down to the floor and use a block if necessary to keep your back flat.

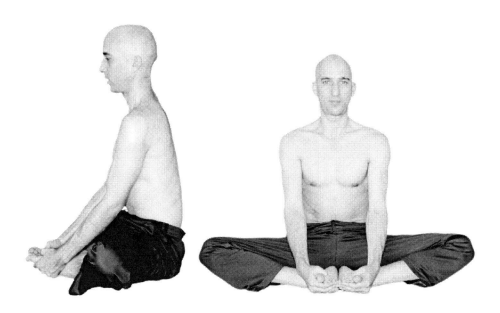

Cobbler's Pose with flat back

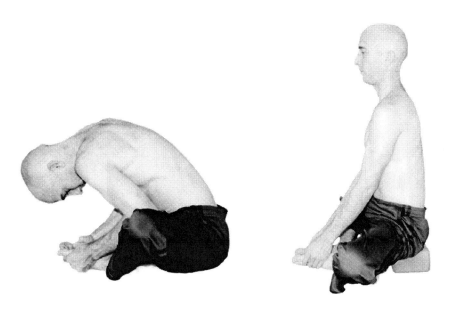

Avoid forward bend and rounding back   Use Block

Lying Down Poses

Happy Baby, Half Happy Baby and Seated Leg Behind the Head should all be avoided. Perform the "figure 4" hip opener instead with your back flat on the mat.

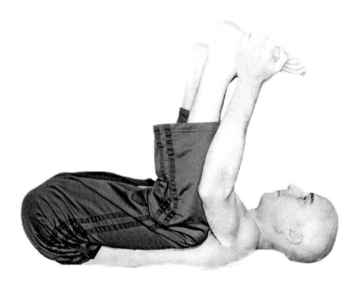

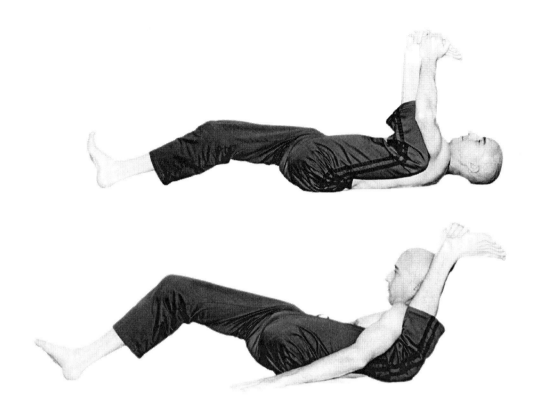

Avoid the above

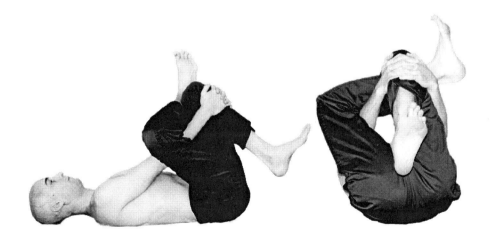

Substitute – "Figure 4" Pose

Plow

Plow can safely be performed if you keep your legs wide apart, your knees bent and you are very gentle. Otherwise avoid Plow and substitute the straight leg pull.

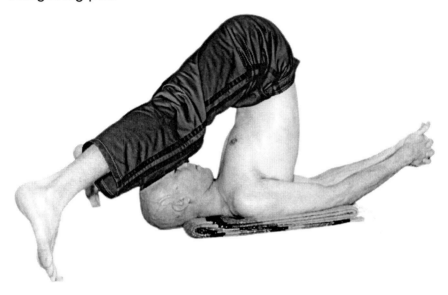

Wide Leg Plow – Back must be flat

Knees to Chest

Perform this pose with one leg at a time and keep your back perfectly flat on your mat.

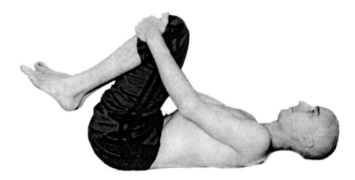

Avoid

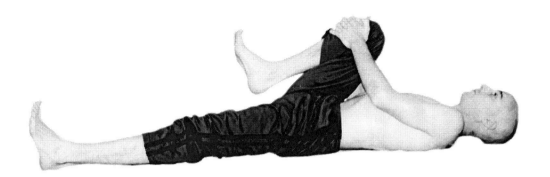

Safe Alternative

Savasana

Make sure to use a pillow or bolster to support your knees in this pose.

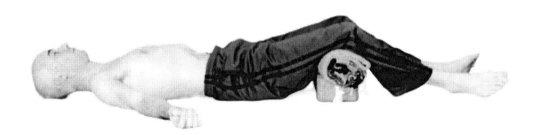

Chapter Twenty One— Strengthening

Now that you have learned how to lengthen your hamstrings and protect your back from injury, you need to strengthen your core to provide muscular support for your back. This will improve your posture, alleviate stress on your back and support a Healing Environment.

Here are a few simple movements that you should be doing in your practice.

Push-Up or Push up on knees

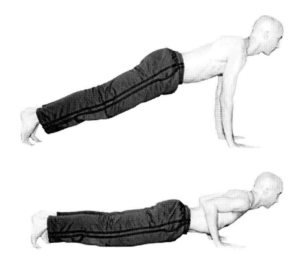

Note: You may also hold plank if you are not yet strong enough for push ups

Side Plank

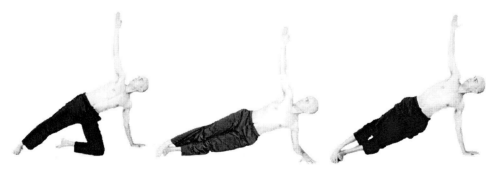

Beginner   Intermediate Options

Superman

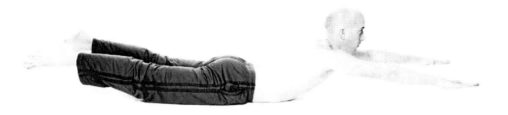

Crunches

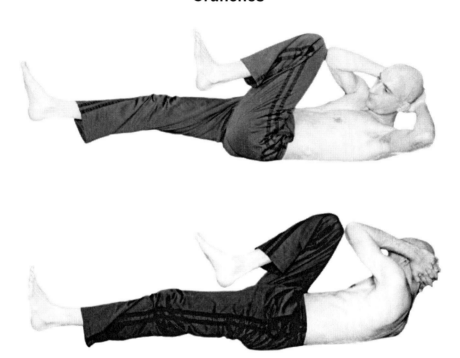

If these poses are not called out at your yoga class, you should do them at the end. As your strength increases, you should try to repeat these in a circuit at least three times. These movements will be very beneficial to the health of your back.

Chapter Twenty Two — Back Bending

As discussed in earlier, back-bending is generally safe for people with back injuries. The one caveat is that the bending must be performed in a manner that minimizes compression on the back. This is done by expanding the arch of the bend by lifting the chest and rotating the pelvis away from the bend (see illustration). Remember, back-bending is really a front stretch.

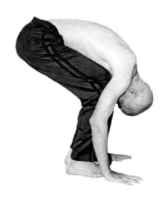

Chapter Twenty Three — Seated Position without Stressing Back

Most yoga classes include some seated meditation. In many cases this position is held for an extended period. If you have tight hips, this position can be quite stressful on your lower back and uncomfortable. If you can only flatten your back by using an extreme amount of muscular effort an adjustment should be made. Sit on blocks or a cushion. You will enjoy meditation much more, and your back will thank you.

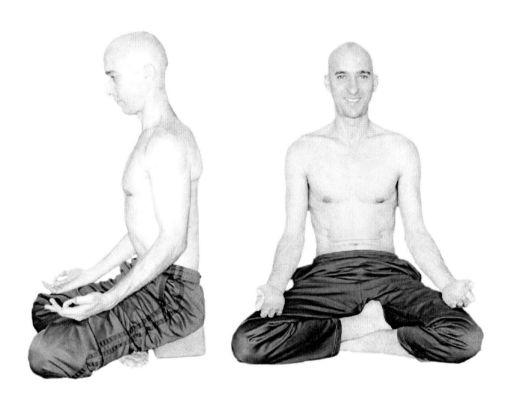

Chapter Twenty Four — Your Own Practice

Thus far we have focused on how to modify your practice in a yoga class to eliminate back pain. Attending yoga class is fun and can make your practice more enjoyable. On the other hand, practicing on your own can result in a deep personal experience where you can tailor your practice to fit your particular needs without the constraints of a class setting. You also have the flexibility of practicing whenever and wherever you like. It is my hope that you will be able to do both. To that end, I will share with you my power yoga series modified for healing back pain.

Opening Sequence

Cat-Cow Flow

Neutral
Align your hands underneath your shoulders, knees underneath your hips

Cow
Inhale, drop your belly, look up

Cat
Exhale, round your back like a cat look at your belly

Repeat 3-4 times

Downdog
Exhale, Alternately, bend your knees & shake your head yes & no
5 BREATHS

One Legged Downdog

Inhale your right leg up, square your hips
3-4 BREATHS

Downdog
Exhale your Right leg down

Inhale your Left leg up, square your hips
3-4 BREATHS

Downdog
Exhale your Left leg down

Kneeling
1 BREATH

One Legged Downdog with Hip Opener

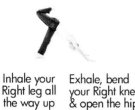 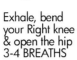

Inhale your
Right leg all
the way up

Exhale, bend
your Right knee
& open the hip
3-4 BREATHS

Downdog
Exhale your
Right leg down

Inhale your
Left leg all the
way up

Exhale, bend
your Left knee &
open the hip
3-4 BREATHS

Downdog
Exhale your
Left leg down

Kneeling
1 BREATH

Downdog
5 BREATHS

Vinyasa Flow - The 4 Steps To Downdog

1. Plank *
Inhale
Up

2. Plank
Exhale
Down

3. Cobra
Inhale
Look up
See instructions
on page ___

4. Downdog
Exhale
Look at navel

* Options:
1. Stay in plank top or bottom for 3 BREATHS
2. Drop to your knees and do 3 push-ups
3. Do 3 regular push ups

Sun Salutation A

Moving Meditation - Merging breath and movement - 2-4 Rounds

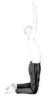

Raised Mountain Inhale, your arms up, look up

Lower your arms and Exhale

Come to neutral position on hands and knees Inhale, look up half way, open your heart

Plank Exhale, step your feet back lower down to the ground

Cobra Inhale, look up

   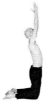

Downdog Exhale, Look at the Navel Stay for 5 BREATHS

Come to neutral position on hands and knees Inhale, look up half way, open your heart

Kneeling with arms at your sides Exhale

Raised Mountain Inhale your arms up, look up

Mountain Exhale your arms down

Sun Salutation B

Moving Meditation - Merging breath and movement - 2-4 Rounds

   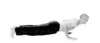

Raised Mountain Inhale, your arms up, look up

Lower your arms and Exhale

Come to neutral position on hands and knees Inhale, look up half way, open your heart

Plank Exhale, step your feet back lower down to the ground

Cobra Inhale, look up

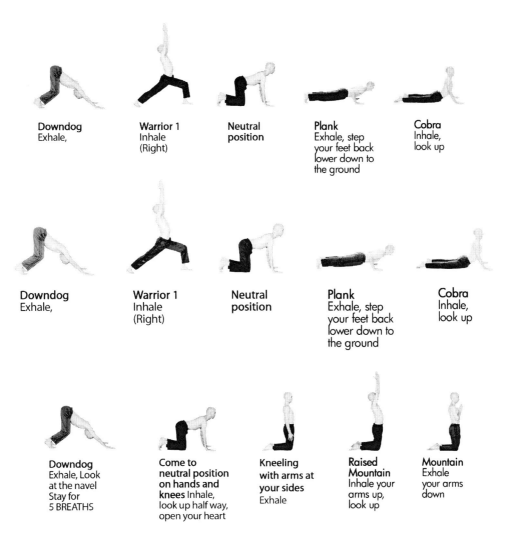

Downdog
Exhale,

Warrior 1
Inhale
(Right)

Neutral position

Plank
Exhale, step your feet back lower down to the ground

Cobra
Inhale, look up

Downdog
Exhale,

Warrior 1
Inhale
(Right)

Neutral position

Plank
Exhale, step your feet back lower down to the ground

Cobra
Inhale, look up

Downdog
Exhale, Look at the navel Stay for 5 BREATHS

Come to neutral position on hands and knees Inhale, look up half way, open your heart

Kneeling with arms at your sides
Exhale

Raised Mountain
Inhale your arms up, look up

Mountain
Exhale your arms down

Standing

Warrior II / Side Angle Series

Step your Right foot up in between your hands

Warrior I
Inhale
Look at your hands

Warrior II
Exhale,
Look to your front hand
3-5 BREATHS

Side Angle A
Look at your top hand

Warrior II

Side Angle B
Look at your top hand
3-5 BREATHS

Complete on the right, do a vinyasa then repeat on the left.

Vinyasa Flow

1. Plank
Inhale Up

2. Plank
Exhale Down

3. Cobra
Inhale, look up

4. Downdog
Exhale, look
to your navel

Vinyasa Flow

    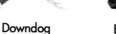

1. Plank
Inhale Up

2. Plank
Exhale Down

3. Cobra
Inhale, look up

4. Downdog
Exhale, look
to your navel

(Optional) Side Crow

Side Crow
(Right / Left)

OR
Replacement
Options

Downdog

Boat

Vinyasa Flow

1. Plank
Inhale Up

2. Plank
Exhale Down

3. Cobra
Inhale, look up

4. Downdog
Exhale, look
to your navel

Middle Sequence

Camel

1. Camel
Hands on your
lower back
3-5 BREATHS

2. Camel
One hand on
your heel
3-5 BREATHS

3. Camel
Both hands
on your heels
3-5 BREATHS

Superhero Series - Cobra (Sacra - Iliac Therapy)

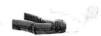

Superhero Variation 1
Inhale your arms & legs up , look up
3-5 BREATHS

REST
on
the
floor

Superhero Variation 2
Grasp your hands behind your back
(a) Inhale your legs apart

(b) Exhale your legs together

REST
on
the
floor

Cobra
Look up

Repeat 3-5 times

Peacock

**Peacock
Preparation**
Place your palms on the floor, fingers facing back

**Peacock
Option 1**
Place your head on the floor and extend the legs back
3-5 BREATHS

**Peacock
Option 2**
Lift the head off the floor
3-5 BREATHS

**Peacock
Option 3**
Lift the legs and keep your head off the floor
3-5 BREATHS

(Optional) Forearm Stand

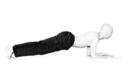

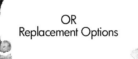

OR
Replacement Options

OR

Optional Plank
(Forearm Stand Prep)
3-5 BREATHS

**Optional
Forearm Stand**

*(At the wall or for
Advanced students ONLY)*

Downdog

Boat

Bound Angle /Reverse Table

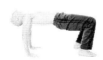

Bound Angle
Look ahead

Reverse Table
Look Up
3-5 BREATHS

Seated Spinal Twist

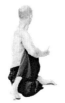 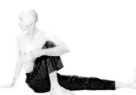

Right/Left

Spinal Twist
Option 1
Bent knee
Twist and look back
3-5 BREATHS

Spinal Twist
Option 2
Straight leg
Twist and look back
3-5 BREATHS

Core Boost : Boat

3 Rounds Up (Sets of 5 Breaths : Legs bent)
2 Rounds Down (Sets of 5 Breaths : Legs extended)
Optional 1 - 2 sets of Crunches (10 in each set at the end)

Boat

Pigeon

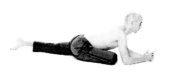 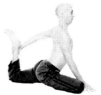

Pigeon
Look down
5 BREATHS OR MORE

(Optional)
King Pigeon
Variation
3-5 BREATHS

Savasana

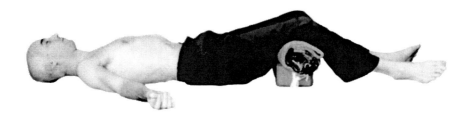

Chapter Twenty Five — Final Thoughts

Even if you have had chronic and severe lower back pain for years, you can become pain free if you incorporate the poses and practices outlined in this book into your daily life. Equally important to the physical discipline, however, is your mental attitude.

One of the most insidious things that prevents us from healing and from experiencing peace in your lives is the victim mentality. It is absolutely critical to liberate yourself from this pernicious presence in your life. It is critical that you no longer identify yourself as someone with back pain, or as someone who is the victim of back pain.

Remember that everything happens for a reason and that lessons learned from the experience of back pain are very valuable.

Feel gratitude always. If you have back pain, it means you have a living body. Give thanks! Your pain will be gone soon and when it leaves, don't look for it ever again. Just let it go!

Continue your yoga practice after you are pain free. Many poses that were once beyond your reach can be resumed once you have lived pain free for a year or two.

Get ready... now to enjoy your pain-free life.

Notes:

Notes:

Notes:

Notes:

CPSIA information can be obtained at www.ICGtesting.com
Printed in the USA
BVOW061236300113

311954BV00004B/356/P